The *Law of*
Attraction
GAME BOOK

28 Days Of *Love*

SPARK your Self Worth With
Daily Inspiration
IGNITE Your Self Esteem and
Self Confidence With FUN!

The Law of Attraction

Game Book

28 Days of Love

With a sprinkle of Ho'oponopono

Priya Khajuria

Joyful Life Mastery Books

JOYFUL LIFE MASTERY BOOKS

For information about special discounts for bulk purchases, please contact Joyful Life Mastery at JoyfulLifeMastery@gmail.com.

Artwork and concept by Priya Khajuria
ISBN 978-1-7753295-1-0

Sign up for the Newsletter at:

http://tinyurl.com/yyykdouo or www.JoyfulLifeMastery.com

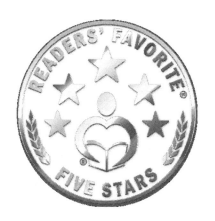

WINNER

CANADA BOOK AWARDS

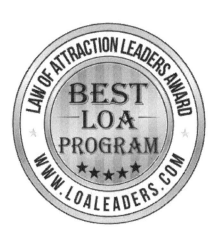

PRAISE:

MARISSA STAPLEY, BEST-SELLING AUTHOR, *Things to Do When It's Raining*

"Wonderfully enlightening. I just loved this book. Khajuria's writing style is inspiring, kind and gently persuasive. It feels like having a conversation with a good friend and contained many lessons about manifesting and living my best life that I'm going to carry with me. Highly recommend!"

JOSHUA CINTRON, AUTHOR & PUBLISHER, *Upon a Moonlight Kiss*

"The material in this book is life changing. This book is a system, a way of life."

PHILIPPA SETTELS, OWNER & FOUNDER of B green

"The Law of Attraction Game Book 28 days of Love' is a delight to read! As adults surrounded by responsibilities, we tend to forget to play sometimes! This gem of a book is the perfect way to start having a little more fun in life and brings the LOA front and center with joy, love and light."

READER'S FAVOURITE (5 STARS)

"...As I read through this little gem of a book, I was struck by the imagination and love of life that went into each day's offering. The first day's subject alone had me thinking about things in an entirely new and positive light... Law of Attraction Game Book: 28 Days of Love is most highly recommended."

AMAZON UK (5 STARS)

"I love this book. I am really enjoying the daily tasks, I look forward every day to see what is ahead for the day. I feel this book is making me appreciate my body and character. I have read lots of books on the law of attraction but this one really holds my interest, it is refreshingly different, this is a book I will read over and over again until I feel I understand the tasks fully."

To my wonderful parents, whose love supercharged my life.

To my beautiful sister, whose love brings light even into
the darkest of times.

To my gorgeous husband, whose love is all-embracing.

To my strong, powerful, brilliant and beautiful daughters,
…the wonders of my life.

"Appreciation and self-love are the most important tools that you could ever nurture. Appreciation of others, and the appreciation of yourself is the closest vibrational match to your Source Energy of anything that we've ever witnessed anywhere in the Universe."

ABRAHAM HICKS

TABLE OF CONTENTS

PART 1 – 28 DAYS OF LOVE

PART 2 – THE DAILY POWER RITUAL

INTRODUCTION: WHY EVERYTHING STARTS WITH YOU

"Your beliefs become your thoughts,
Your thoughts become your words,
Your words become your actions,
Your actions become your habits,
Your habits become your values,
Your values become your destiny."
GANDHI

Welcome, beautiful Soul!

You are about to embark on a journey that will help you rediscover and unlock the greatness within.

You'll start in a fun and lighthearted way, and then move into richly layered exercises.

Not only will you be astounded at what you discover, you'll also lock in your amazing revelations by creating a simple, daily power ritual at the end of this Game.

Before we start, there is something you should know...

Although *28 Days of Love* was created to be playful, **the exercises in this Game Book will change your life**.

- The way you perceive yourself will change.

- Your self-talk will improve exponentially.

- The way you connect with other people will change.

- Your perception of life will change to one of wonder and increasing delight.

You will come out of this Game stronger within, and more powerful that you can foresee. And this is only the beginning.

This book is based on a real-life Game that was played in my Law of Attraction Facebook Group, with the most heartwarming results. Here's a little bit about the wonderful people who played and who love these Law of Attraction Games. Perhaps you may find yourself relating to them in some or many ways...

They're all ages and from different backgrounds. But most are artists, creatives or lightworkers who juggle traditional and entrepreneurial jobs, family, and other close relationships. They have big dreams, and during an average day may flip from focus to overwhelm.

They want to know how to navigate life in the best way possible, and they move through feeling bewildered to questioning to inspired - and back again. They're philosophical with an open mind and heart, and they question anything that doesn't make sense.

They're sweetness and light – yet they love a good old action movie and don't mind a little "language" at times. They're comfortable accepting and allowing strong emotions so they can release them in a healthy way. They're just a wonderfully big contradiction.
There's simply no putting them in a box!

Players embarking on this little voyage of self-discovery found that it was often a challenge at the start to look for lovable aspects about themselves – but the challenge was well worth it!

Before we start, let's step back a little and look at the landscape...

Everything we experience in life is perceived through filters. Some of these filters include the way we were brought up, our world views, our cultural and social background, our opinions and our life experiences. Many of these filters are rooted deep within our past which colors how we "live" in the present. And how we "live" in the present then projects a specific filter on our future.

Pain and suffering, or beautiful and profound experiences - all are stored as memories in the subconscious mind which affects our current beliefs. The subconscious mind directs most of our conscious activities. It also affects the direction our minds will tend to take.

In other words, **our past experiences guide us towards a habitual way of thinking.**

We translate our memories into stories and then flesh them out with a certain context. We believe it was a good, neutral or bad experience. And with time and repetition, when we come across similar situations or experiences, our mind redirects itself again towards that original context, deepening the connection.

A habitual way of thinking – whether negative or positive – automatically draws and directs our attention and energy away from the present moment.
Meaning that in many ways, **we are unconsciously living our life on repeat**.

Ironic, isn't it?

We unintentionally create our future based on the past, by projecting past filters onto the future - but in *this moment*.

The present moment is all we ever have in hand. Our power is not in the past or the future. **Our power exists right now.**

Is our past pointless? No, because everything from your past has contributed to the person you are today. And right now, in this very moment, you are fabulous.

Let that sink in for a minute...

Not "perfect" (there's no such thing anyway, thank goodness)
But Wonderful.

Perhaps you're looking at the word *wonderful* and thinking "well, I'm not there yet."

Or perhaps, you're thinking about your so-called flaws. If so, I get it. We all do it. We focus immediately on weaknesses we seem to have, or a body area we aren't too happy with. Or perhaps you're thinking about dreams you want to attain, milestones you're yearning to reach, and don't feel "complete" yet.

Want to know a secret? All of us feel this way, at different times, and for various things. The first thing to do now...is be kind to yourself. Gently release any judgements about yourself that arise, at least for the duration of the Game. As you play - and with repeat games – you'll find it so much easier to let go of self-criticism.

Part of the problem is that we tend to compare ourselves to others. Or we try to figure out whether we fit the standard of self as it "should" be. That "should" being defined by cultural or religious norms, or determined by any other group that purports to lead the standards that one should aspire to.

When we don't live up to the "shoulds" for whatever reason, we tend to fall prey to self-criticism and feelings of unworthiness.

But you, are quite simply, YOU.
Unique and wondrous.

Of course, there are inner shadows that you don't want to bypass. And you may be in the process of working through deep healings and making life changes.

Gently allow yourself to play anyway. This Game is all about playfully allowing in clarity and focus through fun and simplicity. As you play, you'll naturally feel lighter - and indeed - you'll allow in the light itself. It's through this awakening light that your shadows can gently be accepted and painful thoughts released, so healings can occur.

With this Game, you'll intentionally set aside a block of time each day to play. You will really and truly recognize and appreciate yourself on different levels AND from the very specific contexts of self-love and self-worth.

If you're new to the Law of Attraction, it is a Universal Law that states that you attract into your life the overriding essence and direction of what you focus on.

Have you ever read the quote "thoughts become things"?

This quote sums up the various stages in the Law of Attraction cycle. The cycle moves from your beliefs, feelings and thoughts through your focus and clarity into inspired action to eventually manifesting your experiences.

Clarity is one of the secret keys to successfully flowing with the Law of Attraction. The clearer you are about anything, the more life you bring to whatever you're thinking about or observing.

This Game guides you through an inner journey of self-discovery that is both light-hearted and transformative. When real-life players made the time to get really clear with their answers, not only did it uplift their moods almost instantly, it had a profound radiating effect outwards to others in their lives.

This Game invites you to set aside your inner critic and truly appreciate yourself!

In the next chapter, I'll show you how to play this Game. There are two main Game plays and you can customize them as you desire.

I promise that if you play this Game every day, you'll be astounded. You will recognize just how valuable and worthy you really are, and much, much more. You won't need to wait 28 days to see or feel the effects, you'll start experiencing them from the very first day!

As you play, you'll move **away** from thinking things like: *How on earth am I wonderful? No one else seems to think so...My life never seems to work out the way I want it, etc.*

Instead, you'll move **towards**: *Oh wow, why haven't I noticed this about myself before? I really AM kind of wonderful!*

How do you connect being "wonderful" with self-love? Well, when you acknowledge all that is wonderful about yourself, you enhance your own sense of lovability. You see for *yourself* that you are lovable.

Your level of self-awareness and where you decide to direct your focus affects many things. It affects the relationships you experience, your jobs or career and the way your day plays out. How you react to people and events evolves from this self-awareness.

This Game Book will increase your self-awareness along with your self-love. Connecting with your inner self in a new and enhanced loving way *strengthens* your inner self-power, your self-confidence and self-awareness. The Law of Attraction then ensures that you attract more of the same.

Try a little experiment with me...

Think of the word "love" and scan your body to sense how it reacts. In this case, I'm talking about pure, platonic love. Think of a kitten or a child; something or someone you love with complete abandon and joy. Visualize them right now. Feel the emotions connected to them.

Do you feel yourself smiling?
Perhaps, the muscles around your eyes are relaxing?
Do you feel softer, more expansive?

Can you feel all these sensations and more in your body?

Love is *expansion*. The universe is based on expansion. When we connect with each other in a spirit of love or joy, we feel expansive.

Love is *connection*.
With ourselves.
With each other.

When we love, we are aligned in that very moment with the power and energies of the Universe.
We are plugged in!
And we naturally radiate that love outwards, which is such an "attractive" quality in all ways!

The problem is, sometimes we get caught up looking for love everywhere else but from ourselves. And societal and cultural conditioning can often muddy up the idea of self-love by comparing it to selfishness or conceit. No wonder our society suffers from so many self-worth issues!

Self-love doesn't mean trying to fit in and hide your voice.
Self-love isn't about blindly following everything you've been told and taught.
And self-love doesn't mean repressing your emotions to "be nice."

It's not selfish to love or appreciate yourself.

It's not conceited to be proud of something you've accomplished.

When you love and appreciate yourself, you give tacit permission to others to do the same. You inspire them. You free them. And you appreciate the accomplishments of others from a place of power within.

There is no competition between serving others and loving ourselves. In fact, when we truly love ourselves, we are far more *authentic* in how we serve others and connect with each other.

Self-love is the understanding, acceptance and appreciation of yourself. It is a form of deep gratitude to the Universe for the gift of YOU to this world.

Self-love boosts self-esteem.
And self-esteem ramps up self-confidence.

Self-love, self-esteem and self-confidence are the most **powerful** building blocks in life! They affect your choices in the moment and for the future.

They also affect everyone around us and *their* lives. They affect how you process your past and what you choose to release or treasure (there's no judgement or wrong answer for this).

But...how do you boost self-love?
You simply practice a little bit every day.

We often confuse self-care with self-love. Self-care is not the same as self-love, although it is part of it. Self-care involves taking care of ourselves on all levels. We may buy lovely clothes, go to the spa, go on vacation, eat and drink well, make time for relaxation, etc. etc. but *care* is only one aspect of *love*.

LOVE is positive and joyful, focused attention and acceptance in this very moment.

SELF-LOVE is making the time and giving yourself space to notice your great qualities (giving yourself the attention). And accepting yourself AS YOU ARE in this moment.

This energy propels itself from the "now" into the next moment and the moment after - it springs into the energy of our "future." This attraction and expansion of love will bring in more to love!

In this Game, you will start the FIRE of self-love, by reclaiming your attention towards YOU. From Day 1, you will really, truly notice what is lovable about yourself.

This Game is for you...

- If you compare yourself to others.
- If you fear you're not good enough.
- If you often doubt yourself.
- If you feel guilty when you stand up for yourself.
- If you feel that the rest of the world seems to be having more fun.

I invite you to take a little time every day to appreciate yourself - this is *your life,* my friend.

Know that you are LOVABLE and WORTHY.

Always.

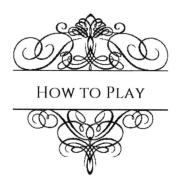

HOW TO PLAY

A s you play this Game, you will contemplate aspects that you love about yourself, your life experiences and your surroundings.

The point of the Game is to gently and consistently draw your attention to what you love. And by the Law of Attraction, as you continue this habit, you create a strong momentum which brings you more to discover and love!

The Game involves about 5-15 minutes of your time per day (or more, when you get really into it!). You'll receive a little question to contemplate and a little exercise to complete. Ponder the question for as long as you can during the day, even after you've played. Look for insights and aha's.

Have you ever watched a movie for the second (or third) time and noticed things you missed the first time?

13

You can replay this Game anytime you like and when you do, you'll discover even more to love!

The regular Game play is introduced each day with the **PlayBites** – these are short and sweet game plays at the beginning of each chapter. The Game content then dives deeper into each topic and includes additional exercises called the **Advanced Game Plays**. You can choose to keep the Game light by using only the PlayBites, or you can go deeper with the additional content and the Advanced Game Plays.

In a few of the Advanced Game Plays, you'll use two of the most powerful mantras in Ho'oponopono, which is a new take on an ancient Hawaiian metaphysical healing technique. The metaphysical applications of Ho'oponopono itself are extremely layered and deeply spiritual. However, for the purposes of this Game, we're going to use just two of the four main mantras to clear and refresh your energy in the context of love and self-love.

You might be tempted to skim through the content first. That's fine – you'll definitely see and feel results just by reading through this book. But to get the most out of this Game, either keep a notebook handy as you play or type your answers in an online document.

You can also use the printable version of the PlayBites called the Playsheets. What's the difference between the PlayBites and the Playsheets? The PlayBites are the content that we played with in the actual live Game. And with only those little prompts and questions, many joyous transformations happened. The Playsheets are a beautiful full page colour version of the PlayBites that you can print and use as your own – write all over them, make them yours. The link is near the end of this book – you'll find them with the Bonuses.

Regardless of whether you skim through the book or play in detail, be sure to take the time to think about each question and your answer. Getting your hands and senses right into the Game sends a powerful message to your subconscious that you are making the time to honor yourself.

The PlayBite questions may seem extremely simple at first – that's on purpose, they're meant to be fun and bring back your focus to the beautiful soul that is YOU. You'll notice that each day's Game play is moving intentionally in specific directions, and each day builds upon the one before. From the inside to the outside, from lighter to deeper, and through intentions and time.

At the end of the Game, I'll walk you through a powerful daily practice that you will create called THE DAILY POWER RITUAL. The Ritual takes only 5 minutes a day and will lock in all that you discover during the Game. When used regularly, this Ritual will energize anything you choose to manifest.

When you strengthen your inner core with love and confidence, you begin to choose desires that are truly appealing to you. And this changes your focus and what you manifest into your life.

As I mentioned, it is my promise to you that each time you play this Game, you'll find even **more** to appreciate about yourself. Each time, you'll be unravelling more, noticing more, enjoying and engaging more of your qualities.

Your focus on your positive aspects continues to build your self-acceptance and your self-esteem. All of which supercharges your self-confidence.

And that beautiful energy then radiates out and attracts matching people, situations and life experiences.

This Game will open your heart to yourself in the most astonishing and profoundly beautiful ways.

When you play, write down whatever springs to mind right away.

We're not going to look at any limiting beliefs.
We're not going to try to "fix" anything.
We're just going to play and flow.

Ready?

YOU'LL NEED:

- A smile
- 5-15 minutes a day
- Nice notepaper or a notebook (or the printed Playbook)
- A pen that you love

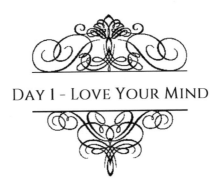

DAY 1 - LOVE YOUR MIND

10 THINGS YOU LOVE ABOUT YOUR MIND:

Your mind is your ethereal chariot.

Your Will holds the reins.

What do you LOVE your mind to dwell

upon and think about?

Ready....go!

Y our mind can be your greatest friend or enemy. It can travel down paths and corridors with or without intention.

Indeed, your mind - how you think and where you direct your thoughts - may be one of the greatest challenges in life to master.

Consistent thoughts and the way we translate life experiences into memories lead to subconscious beliefs. Which in turn may bubble up as repetitious thought patterns that we often catch ourselves experiencing in mid-action.

It is guess-timated that we think anywhere from 70,000 - 600,000 thoughts a day! And most of these are repetitive and negative.

The Law of Attraction ensures that we primarily see and experience things that align with our beliefs. So try your best to be conscious and aware of your daily thought patterns so you can steer them in the direction of what you want, appreciate or enjoy.

There's nothing wrong with contemplating something that isn't working well for you. In fact, these trigger situations are referred to by Abraham-Hicks as *contrast*, and they can be the springboard towards creating change. It's when we stay stuck in these thoughts or we don't act, that we continue to allow our thoughts to travel in an unwanted direction and then they begin to eat away at us.

As love and relationship coach Lisa Marie Hayes says, "We tend to believe our own thoughts even when they don't prove themselves to be accurate." Being stuck in this type of thought pattern also begins to attract similar thoughts and a negative momentum is created.

So if you're experiencing a job, living or other situation that is not ideal for you, begin by clarifying what you *would* like and start focusing and moving towards those new scenarios every day.

Abraham-Hicks states that "when you hold a thought for 17 seconds – only 17 seconds, another thought that is vibrationally the same joins that thought. And after 68 seconds if you are able to maintain a momentum, you'll have true movement in your vibration.

"As you're in your "now" and you are thinking about those 17 second explosions and you are making an effort to lean in the direction of what you're wanting - now you're in control in every moment and 30 days of that "*loose awareness*" cleans your vibration up on so many subjects that people who are watching you would hardly recognize you as the same person in terms of what's beginning to flow into your experience."

You can apply the Abraham-Hicks quote here to any pattern of thought – or as a start towards any desire you'd like to manifest.

However, for the purpose of this Game, know that each 17 seconds you spend feeling and expressing love for yourself will simply attract a greater awareness of how lovable you are!

So, back to your mind...you have certain thought patterns that work very well for you now. You have attracted some wonderful things into your life because of where and how you focused your mind.

And sometimes you just like to think about things that make you happy.

What are some of these things?

Advanced Game Play:

For 5 days, simply be aware of your thoughts. How do you do that when there are roughly 60,000 thoughts running through our minds a day?

By noticing your feelings. Your feelings are emanating from the types of thoughts that are running through your mind, many on autopilot and most of them reactive and automatic.

Here's an easy way to do this:

1. Set up a Calendar reminder on your phone or on your computer (I use my Google calendar).

2. Your reminder should be set up 3 times, spread out through the day.

3. At each prompt, scan your feelings in that moment. Ask yourself *what am I feeling right now? Anticipation? Fun? Joy? Boredom? Annoyance, or something else not-so-good?*

4. If you feel good, ask yourself *what have I been thinking or doing to feel this?* Get right into the details, enjoy it. Expand it for as long as you can.

5. If the feelings are heavy or meh, once again ask yourself *what have I been thinking about, to feel this way?*

6. Then pull out two small sheets of paper and label one DO and the other RELEASE. Think about what has been leading your thoughts into heavier feelings and add them to one of the two lists as follows: For something you can change, add it to the DO list. For something that you really cannot change due to the circumstances, your choice in the present, or other reasons, note them down on the RELEASE list.

7. Take action on the DO list. By taking action, you're saying to yourself that you're in charge of your actions and will do what you must to right things. This completes the cycle, and will result in higher feelings of self-belief.

8. Rip up the RELEASE list. By ripping it up, you're releasing these items to the Universe – a higher Power – to resolve. This creates mental space by releasing what is effectively mental clutter.

9. Important: After ripping up the RELEASE list, immediately switch your attention to a visual of

something joyful as it helps direct your thoughts away from the unwanted and which you have now decided to release. i.e, look at a pet's picture, or an ocean or mountain scene – anything that will capture your attention for a brief time. This completes the cycle - a different cycle from the DO list - but it also signals to yourself that you have addressed what is not working for you, and switched your attention to something that feels better. This results in greater feelings of peace and the ability to *make peace* with the present.

Day 2 - Compliments from Others

10 Things Others Compliment You For:

Genuine compliments from others are 3D holographic versions of living affirmations.

Your joyful self-expressions are transmitted and received by others with delight.

What are you celebrated for?
Anything goes.
Ready....go!

F or this exercise, think back to sincere compliments you've received in the past. They may be related to your personality, appearance, or perhaps they're about something you've said or done.

Maybe you truly inspired someone one day, or your smile and a few words were enough to set a wonderful butterfly effect in motion for others. Or maybe you received sincere compliments on your personal qualities.

Genuine compliments are a form of beautiful energy flowing back to you. They have been generated by your own energy that you put out there into the world. Compliments are also a lovely way to see your qualities and other positive "life aspects" through the eyes of others.

Sometimes it can be difficult to receive compliments. Think back a little to your reactions when you receive one. Do you tend to shrug them off? Or do you feel modest and humble about compliments and find it difficult to accept them?

Accepting and really *seeing and feeling* a compliment engages your focus and attention on wonderful things about yourself that are appreciated or noticed by others. And it also enhances the sense of your own contribution to our connected Universe.

In today's exercise, let's celebrate all that you're complimented for. Make a list of 10 recent compliments and don't be shy!

Advanced Game Play:

Give someone a sincere compliment today.

If you really want to ramp up some major high-vibes, set up a daily Calendar reminder for the next 30 days. Add each of these into the Calendar:

- Find something about yourself to compliment.
- Tell your child about something lovely you noticed in them today.
- Tell your spouse about something wonderful you noticed in them today.
- Thank your colleague for something and let them know 1 thing you appreciate about them.
- Give a stranger a sincere compliment at the grocery store.
- Do you take the bus or train to work? Give someone you normally see there a compliment and watch their eyes shine!
- Compliment your pet! They'll certainly understand your vibration as you say it!
- Call your mother or father and give them a sincere compliment at the end of your chat.
- Text your brother or sister and give them a compliment.
- Post a compliment on your friend's Facebook page.

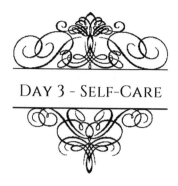

DAY 3 - SELF-CARE

10 FAVOURITE SELF-CARE TREATS:

Self-care is a powerful message you send to your subconscious - that you are worth it.

Self-care is an integral part of self-love.
What are your favorite ways to indulge in self-care?

And which are you planning on doing today?
Ready....go!

S elf-care is essential to wellbeing. It's a necessary practice to soothe, refresh and reenergize your body, mind and spirit. For many busy parents, self-care can fall by the wayside from time to time.

Take a moment to think through your daily schedule and lifestyle and honestly assess it. Do you tend to get caught up in your day and put self-care on a back-burner? Or maybe overdo one or two aspects (i.e. mind and spirit) and throw the third aspect out of balance?

It's so important to be really honest about what you love in terms of self-care and then add it in to your day however you can. Always aim for all three aspects (mind, body and spirit) and if you don't have a chance to incorporate them in a given day, reassure yourself that you'll tend to it tomorrow.

Be kind to yourself as well, it's quite normal to let these fall through the cracks when you're busy juggling many things, just aim to gently add them in again, a little at a time, however you can.

For fun, make a master list of your favorite self-care treats in the Advanced Game Play. Leave the list by the side of your bed so you can glance at it each day.

Advanced Game Play:

Create a list under each heading: *Body, Mind, and Spirit.*

For example, under *Body*, note down all the things you love to do to refresh your body.

Do you enjoy massages?
How about a spa visit?
Do you love mani-pedis?
Maybe you enjoy taking a relaxing walk in nature?
Perhaps you have fun when you visit the gym, or take a dance class?

Write down everything you can, then do the same for *Mind* and *Spirit*. Some items may overlap and that's okay.

In my case, I love to read uplifting and motivational books each morning to get my mind fresh and ready for the day. In the evenings, I love to wind down with a glass of wine and about 20 minutes from a historical romance – usually involving Scottish lairds or Victorian ladies. My husband gets a kick out of the novel names (titles like *Unlaced by The Highland Duke* or *The Viscount's Lady*). When the weather is good, I usually go out for a walk on the lakefront to re-energize all aspects of me. Write down what *you* love, and don't judge any of it!

Once your list is complete, look at your list every day and ask yourself: *Which of these would I like to do today?*

And then do them.

Day 4 - Cool things About You

10 Cool Things:

Every day you do something awesome that you may not even notice.
Think about it now...

What did you do yesterday or this past week that you're really proud of?

Anything goes.
Ready....go!

I n this exercise, take a little time to remember several things you've said or done recently that you consider to be pretty awesome.

Now, even though this Game Book is all about the wonderfulness that is you – the questions and the exercises are not intended to be self-centered or narcissistic.

In fact, studies show that most people tend to suffer from the exact opposite self-perception, which is why it is so critical that you really and truly see, feel and understand your worth.

Make a list of your cool aspects and contributions, regardless of who may or may not have noticed them or experienced them. The point of this exercise is for *you* to see and acknowledge them. The easiest way is to start with today.

What have you done today that you're satisfied or excited about? (Ignore anything that is the opposite, we all have them, let them go, focus only on what you really liked).

Perhaps you reached out to a new client. Perhaps you paid a bill, enjoyed a sweet moment with your pet, kissed your kids, completed a task at work in a way that satisfied you, sent a donation, made it to work on time, offered a hug, made a phone call or sent an email to someone who needed it, or accomplished anything else that made you feel really good or just plain satisfied.

There's no ranking system here, nothing that makes one thing better than the other – just note anything at all that you said or did that you're proud of.

How about yesterday?
Last week?

Advanced Game Play:

Now think back – what cool things did you do last month?

Keep going backwards in time like this, jotting down anything and everything you can think of.

Once you're done, read through your list and simply rest in the feeling of all the things you have already achieved and accomplished.

You are awesome!

Day 5 - Love Your Accomplishments

10 Accomplishments:

Sometimes we forget how far we have come in such a short time.
Think back...

What are some of your accomplishments in the last month or year?

Anything goes.
Ready....go!

T his is similar to yesterday's concept but in this exercise look for the "big steps," the strides that you really put a lot of effort into. Look for the creation or manifestation of something that you consider a big jump and that you're exceptionally proud of.

Perhaps you started a new job, wrote a book, learned a new instrument or gained a new skill, moved to a new city or country, created something whether it was an article, a song or a meal from a new recipe. Anything goes here too, so look for and celebrate all you've accomplished so far!

Accomplishments are a wonderful reminder that you successfully brought your desire, intention or goal through all the manifestation steps into reality.

You thought about them and believed that it was possible to achieve or create them. You took action and you flowed with the momentum.

Advanced Game Play:

Which of your accomplishments did you manifest from beginning to end *consciously*? By that I mean, which ones did you see in your mind's eye before or as you started?

Which ones were particularly satisfying to achieve? Why? How did it make you feel about yourself?

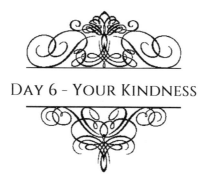

DAY 6 - YOUR KINDNESS

10 KINDNESSES:

When we're kind to others, we often take that for granted.

But your kind words or deeds have an incredible butterfly effect...

What are some ways in which you showed your kind heart recently?
Ready....go!

K indness is imbued with such a loving, gentle energy. Just about everyone responds to kindness – it's sweet, innocent and it connects people together from the heart. Kindness is an outward manifestation of Love.

The thing is, we don't often notice when we're kind to ourselves or someone else. We don't really think about it. Have you done something sweet for someone and then been surprised when they mentioned how kind you were?

I think that one of the reasons for this is that our primary attention is directed towards "not so kind" stories in the news. It's what we're exposed to. Face it, it's mostly the bad stuff that gets reported in the news. And it's all around us! If you're on social media, you'll get the "trending news" pop ups that are almost always negative. Most train and subway stations have those little TV monitors installed that usually show scrolling news clips – and again, almost all of these are negative.

All of this leaves us feeling powerless and vulnerable. Yet, when you observe your day from beginning to end, there may be many small or large kindnesses mixed in. We just don't notice them as much, because they are overridden by the heavier news messages. Over time and without being aware of it, the energy behind constant negative news (or any source of negativity) tends to create an acidity that eats away at our natural state of innocence and openness.

You must be conscious, aware and alert to notice the energy of most media messages because constant repetition of these seep into the subconscious – in fact any type of repetition will.

You must be strong enough to release that from your life in whatever way you can – so that you can focus on where you want to go, what you want to do, be or have.

This doesn't mean that you have to be uninformed about what's going on in the world, just always remind yourself that the bad stuff is but only a part of what's really happening out there. There are people out there, like you and I, sharing kindness freely and often.

When you're kind to someone - whether it's to yourself or someone else - that's no small matter. You have positively impacted the energy of the Universe in that moment!

Kindness, love, innocence, peace, connection – these are our natural states.

You don't have to be religious, spiritual or from any particular cultural, social or economic background to experience and desire these natural states.

In Ho'oponopono, an ancient Hawaiian healing and clearing practice, it is said that mental clutter, chatter, stories, and unpleasant memories prevent us from fully experiencing these natural states of love, innocence and wellbeing on a daily basis.

There are many excellent ways to clear through stuck or unconscious negative states and old stories (for example; Emotional Freedom Technique, affirmations, hypnotherapy, etc.). You can find tons of free EFT videos on YouTube. There are also many wonderful books on Ho'oponopono – you can Google search for Morrna Simeona and Dr. Hew Len. (One of my favorite books on this topic is *Zero Limits* by Dr Joe Vitale). There will be more about Ho'oponopono in this Game book later on.

And now, think back to anything kind you have done recently for yourself or someone else. Maybe you shared kind words, or perhaps you gave a form of support to someone who needed it desperately.

Maybe it was something you did, something you expressed or shared in an email. A hug, a touch, a smile.

The more you bring these memories into your awareness, the more you change your immediate energy field – and you will feel it emotionally.

Advanced Game Play:

Pick a week for this exercise. Do something kind each day. Write down what it was, and how it made you feel.

- Do something kind for a family member.
- Offer a kind word at work.
- Say something kind to a stranger.
- Do something kind for a homeless person.

DAY 7 - QUALITIES OF SOMEONE SPECIAL

10 QUALITIES:

Think about someone in your life who you admire, or who you are close to.

What is that special thing they have? What do you love about them?

Did you know that you have those very qualities, to be able to notice them?   :)
Ready....go!

I n this exercise, think about someone you admire - someone you really look up to. Take a few minutes now to run through several possibilities in your mind.

- It could be someone who is very much in your life already.

- It could be someone you once met.

- It could be someone you've never met in person - perhaps you've read about them, or followed their life story.

- It could even be a historical figure.

Make a list, then pick out one individual who stands out the most to you at this time. Think about all the qualities they have that you really admire and note them down. Come up with at least 10 and keep going if you have more.

Once you're done, read through the list. I want to share something so important with you here...and you probably realize this already.

Everything you wrote down on that list is a quality you already possess.

You are attuned to those qualities, you are attracted to them. And the more you focus on them and think about them, the Law of Attraction will naturally bring you more people, more situations and more events that display these qualities. You'll naturally enhance these qualities even more in your own life. This is one reason daily gratitude journals are so powerful.

Of course, we can apply that to the flip side of the coin, which is why things seem to get worse when we find ourselves stuck in complaint mode.

Some spiritual teachers suggest that you pick one word a day that describes a quality you want to enhance in your life, and just repeat that word many times during the day. Focus on it, contemplate it.

Advanced Game Play:

Here is a fun exercise I do every now and then, when I want to remind myself that we enhance what we focus on. Read it through first so you know what to do, then try it!

Look straight ahead and let your attention relax. Let your vision relax as well.

Then say to yourself "blue" a couple of times while still gazing gently forward. Without turning around to consciously look for blue objects, the most amazing thing will happen without moving your eyes.

Blue items in the room or the area where you are will slowly begin to pop into your peripheral vision.

Now say to yourself "red" or any other color. Red items will now pop up in your peripheral vision and the other colors will sort of fade back a little.

You can try this with objects, such as cars when you're outside, or even textures and senses. I've said things like "sensation" and instantly become aware of the wind against my skin and the feeling of the pavement under my feet.

I once repeated the word "wealth" when I was on a walk, and instantly a plethora of trees around me stood out and so did the marina, everything else fading into the background. As it happens, a marina is considered a sign of prosperity in the ancient energy flow system of Feng Shui!

We are surrounded by countless stimuli and objects, yet our conscious awareness can only take in so much at any one time.

Your attention and focus enhances what is already there within the bigger picture and brings it forward to you more clearly.

Recognizing and contemplating the qualities of whom you admire will enhance those already-existing qualities in yourself.

DAY 8 - A NEW APPRECIATION

NEW APPRECIATION:

Is there something you didn't like about yourself in the past...but you've realized you now LOVE?

List everything you have now come to appreciate!

Ready....go!

One of the most interesting things that happens over time – and with transformational inner work - is that you gain a new appreciation about yourself, especially regarding qualities you might not have liked in the past.

This could be related to your appearance, your skills, your attitudes, your achievements, your quirks, anything really. When we played this Game live, players were surprised and delighted to realize that they now really valued something about themselves that they hadn't before. A lot of this has to do with self-acceptance.

Are there things about yourself that you've really grown into them now but you weren't crazy about these things when you were younger?

Make a list of the following, and note down what you have really and truly come to appreciate about yourself over time, when it comes to these:

- Your values
- Your personality
- Your appearance
- The way you connect with others
- Your skills
- Your habits
- Your preferences and your quirks

Advanced Game Play:

The above exercise involved things you learned to appreciate over time.

In this exercise, you are going to play in the present. Pick a 5-7 day schedule for this.

At the end of each day, think back through the day and jot down anything you appreciate about yourself...

- What are some of things you said today that you appreciate?

- What are some of things you did today that you appreciate?

- Did you redirect heavy thoughts to lighter ones, ones that gave you peace and power?

- What did you offer others today, that you appreciate?

- How were you even more efficient and effective than the day before?

- List other ways that you rocked your day.

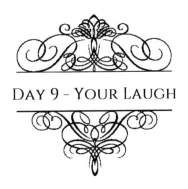

Day 9 - Your Laugh

10 Things You Love About Your Laugh:

Is it the way it sounds?

How it feels?

How and when you laugh?

What makes you laugh?

Ready....go!

T here's a saying you've probably heard: *laughter is the best medicine*. Aside from the obvious benefits of feeling good, there have been many scientific studies on the healing and rejuvenating effects of laughter.

Norman Cousins was a journalist and professor who is probably most famous for curing himself of a debilitating disease by watching funny movies. According to Cousins, ten minutes of laughter in a day resulted in his experiencing 2 hours of pain-free sleep. And according to psychiatrist Dr Kavita Khajuria, "of all the commonly endorsed character strengths, humor contributes most strongly to life satisfaction."

But did you know that not only is laughing great for *you*, it also uplifts and benefits *everyone* in the sphere of your life?

Have you ever had someone smile at you, and for the rest of the day you kept seeing that smile beaming out at you in your mind's eye?

Your smile is a genuine flash of your warmth and humor – it uplifts and engages everyone in its vicinity!

Laughter is even more contagious – it blends a visual of your smile along with sound, boosting the sensory and energetic impact within anyone who hears it. Laughter is a gorgeous boost of heartfelt emotion, and the effects stay with you and anyone on the receiving end.

When you smile or laugh with someone, your energy directly impacts *their* energy field on an even deeper level. For the rest of that day, your laugh has lightened and brightened their mood. When they go home, or come across others during that day, their lighter mood now impacts those whom *they* come across. And the ripple effect just continues from there. You also enhance the physical space you're in – everything is energy!

Along with the benefits of laughter to yourself, you are positively impacting the world around you when you laugh.

Smile and laugh every day - and you change the energy of your world and your life with growing momentum! And that is a gift to the Universe!

Advanced Game Play:

So, let's talk some more about your laugh...

- What makes you giggle? What makes you laugh?

- Which is the last book you read that made you laugh? (Mine was *the 100-Year-Old Man Who Climbed Out the Window and Disappeared by Jonas Jonasson)*

- What was the most recent movie or TV show that made you laugh?

- Which of your friends or relatives laugh the most, and makes you laugh as well?

- There is something fun and funny about yourself that makes you laugh. What is it?

- What do you love about your laugh?

To attract more fun and funny experiences, do more of those things that make you laugh! Spend more time being around those who laugh regularly or who make you laugh.

Or perhaps *you* are the funny one who creates laughter around you...if so, bring more of that into your life and offer it to those around you. Watch that electric energy build and transform into vitality and warm, loving, human connection!

DAY 10 - WHAT YOU LOVE ABOUT YOURSELF

10 THINGS YOU LOVE ABOUT YOURSELF:

There is something about you that is

special and unique.

Not just one thing but many things.

List them.

Ready....go!

N ow we are starting a section of days that many players found challenging at first. This where they felt the most vulnerable, as you may feel too, so the order of days was rearranged to slip these in gently at this stage.

Today you're going to dive into some of the many qualities that make you lovable. There are **a lot**. You may not have noticed all your great qualities but it's imperative that you begin to!

Answer the questions below quickly without thinking too much. If you have difficulty at first, dig deep and look for something good. You'll find it!

- What is unique about you? Stay on this one until you have a good answer!

- There is something very special about you – what is it?

- What is it that you do or say that draws people to you naturally?

- What is your superpower?

- What do people mention that they love, appreciate or enjoy about you? It may be something that you find surprising or not even consider a big deal.

Advanced Game Play:

In this gentle heart-light exercise, you're going to meet with your Higher Self.

Who is your Higher Self? It's the bigger, deeper, inner part of you that is aligned with the vastness of cosmic consciousness. It is your inner Divinity. It is the part of you that remains unaffected by the drama of life, the part that watches over you with boundless love.

Take a deep breath and hold it for a second, then blow it out. Repeat this twice.
Now bring your attention to your heart center. Imagine a luminous white light filling your heart area.

Let it continue to shine and rest there for a few moments. Keep your focus on your heart area and the soft light as it continues to expand.

You may begin to feel a slight surge of energy from your navel upwards.
Send out an intention to engage with your Higher Self. To do this, simply ask to connect and allow the light to flow upwards from your heart and out through the top of your head. You can say a few words out loud if you like, asking your Higher Self to connect with you now.

You may receive images in your mind of your Higher Self with a certain physical form. Or you may receive a sense of warmth or comfort. Your Higher Self *loves* you as you are. Your Higher Self *accepts* you, accepts all that you have experienced and all that you will bring into your future life experience. Ask your Higher Self to help you bring your attention to as many of your lovable qualities as possible.

Now, cast your mind back and reach for loving things you have thought, said or done over the years. Allow your mind to gently sift through memories as they arise. If something unrelated comes up, envision it as a little puff of mist and gently blow it away.

Continue reaching for loving experiences. Love that you have given freely to someone. Love that you have shared with others. Loving thoughts that you have felt. You may feel more surges of energy from your solar plexus and they will feel very joyful. If your mind begins to wander off track a little, simply allow it for a moment and then gently bring your attention back.

Contemplate and rest in this experience for as long as you can, for as long as it feels good. Once you feel fully refreshed, thank your Higher Self. Send love and gratitude to your Higher Self, your past, present and future YOU, and relax.

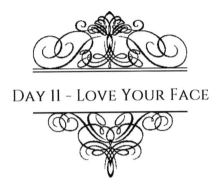

DAY 11 - LOVE YOUR FACE

10 THINGS YOU LOVE ABOUT YOUR FACE:

There is a special sweetness about your

face...something you adore.

Perhaps it's something people mention.

List them and don't be shy!

Ready....go!

T oday's exercise is a little bit more playful - it's all about appreciating your face. Your face is your canvas to the world. Your expressions, your energy - all are visible through your face, your eyes and your expressions.

Your words, your smiles and laughter connect you to other human beings in your physical experience and through your energetic field. Seeing your face makes someone's day!

Think about everything you love about your face. Write down at least 10 things. If you think of more, even better!

Advanced Game Play:

We all have sensitivities about our looks. What you feel is okay. Just remember that the standards of "looks" vary wildly from culture to culture. And our character and personality can override our looks. Our looks can change from day to day, year to year and we can improve it or come to love it – at any time in our life.

In this Game play, we're going to give some massive love to "this face" no matter what the conditions or circumstances.

I highly recommend doing the mirror technique for several days in a row, preferably 21 to 30 days. Louise Hay was the founder of Hay House books and a pioneer in holistic healing education. She credits mirror work as being one of the most profound techniques to learn to love oneself, and it was one that she practiced regularly.

There are many ways to use this technique, but the basic exercise is to look at yourself in the mirror each day and express appreciation. If your day was good, congratulate yourself while looking into your eyes in the mirror.

If it wasn't that good of a day, soothe yourself and give yourself a gentle reminder that tomorrow will be better, and that you will learn from today's experience.

Another easy mirror method is to look at yourself in the mirror in the morning and evening, and just say *I love you* to your reflection. That's it.

This simple act creates a momentum of connection with yourself, and it deepens over time. The more you practice it looking into your eyes, the more you connect with the "you" behind your reflection.

So set up a Calendar reminder, and try the mirror technique daily for as long as it feels good.

Day 12 - Love Your Hair & Head

10 Things You Love About Your Hair:

Touch your hair, really feel it.

Notice the lightplay on it, the shades, the texture.

And if you don't have any hair, notice what you love about your head!

List them!

Ready....go!

Today, you're going to send some love to your hair. No matter what kind of hair you have, or feel you lack, today is the day to send love to every single strand on your head!

Notice the texture...

Is it curly, wavy, straight, fine, thick?
Touch it with your fingers and really *feel* the texture.
What's the color of your hair? The tone, the shade?

If your hair is long, enjoy the sweep of your hair over your shoulders and arms. Enjoy how it feels against your neck and skin.

Now swoosh your hands though your hair like a model on TV! Just do it for fun (no one's watching) and enjoy the sensual feel of your hair running through your fingers.

If your hair is short, rub your hands through it, this way and that, like you would with the fur of a dog or cat. Simply enjoy the feel of it. I'm not comparing your hair to the fur of a pet, what I *am* suggesting is that we allow ourselves to be much freer and more touchy-feely with a pet. Yet why not be just as dear to yourself as a pet would be in every aspect?

Observe the way the light hits your hair. Hold a bit of your hair right now and send waves of love from your heart area to your hair.

And if you happen to be partially or fully bald or shaven, simply send love to every part of your scalp.

Advanced Game Play:

This is an exercise your hair or scalp will love...place your hands on both sides of your head with the fingers pointing towards the back of your head. Place the heels of your palms at the sides of your forehead, over your ears.

Gently apply a little pressure to your scalp and move your palms in a circular manner so that they're gently massaging your head. Move your hands higher up and continue. Then lightly massage the top of your head.

Place your focus and awareness on each area that you're massaging. Now place your hands under your ears and massage the bottom areas of your head.

Once you have completed massaging your head, use the tips of your fingers to lightly tap all over your head in a quick, pressing manner.

Once you are done, your scalp and head should feel freshly energized, yet relaxed.

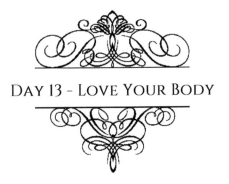

DAY 13 - LOVE YOUR BODY

10 THINGS YOU LOVE ABOUT YOUR BODY:

Sense your body right now.

Feel your heart that beats for you, day and night.

List what you love about your body!

Ready....go!

T oday, you're going to send your entire body some big love just by noticing and appreciating it! Your body is a magnificent vehicle that carries you through this life.

You take about 20,000 breaths a day – your lungs are always working for you.

In one day, your blood travels about 12,000 miles – your heart is always serving you.

Your body produces over 200 billion cells each day and is continuously repairing itself.

Almost every part of your body replaces itself completely at some point in time. Google it, research just how powerful and marvelous your body is. The functions mentioned earlier are just a *fraction* of the miracle that is your body.

Your body is supporting you, day and night. As Law of Attraction coach Jeannette Maw puts it "Every 'symptom' is a healing gesture from the body." **And in the holistic healing world, every symptom is a message from your body.**

Do your conscious thoughts affect your body? Yes, they do and so does your subconscious mind. Your conscious and subconscious thoughts affect what your mind focuses on. They influence your beliefs and direct your mind and in turn affect the actions you take, all of which can affect your body.

Feed your mind positive and healthy thoughts regularly:

- Read something inspiring every morning. 5 minutes is all you need to start a positive flow.

- Unfollow or limit time with people who are consistently negative. You'll feel better, and only they can change the course of their focus and life.

- Limit exposure to the news (it's almost always negative).

- Meditate and breathe deeply each day.

Give importance to how you feel:

- Allow your emotions as they are, and then redirect your attention to something pleasant and desired. It's a mental workout and makes you stronger and more resilient.

- Read something funny.

- Watch something funny.

- Connect often with your higher self, or with your source of inspiration (spirituality, religion, or whatever replenishes and fulfils you).

- Spend time in nature. It's calming and soothing to the spirit.

Set an intention to take charge of your thoughts and feelings from this moment onwards. Allowing yourself to bounce back quickly to something desired and pleasant will create a momentum that will eventually affect your cells (within) and you'll take steps aligned with your beliefs (without).

Advanced Game Play:

Mentally scan your body from head to foot and send thoughts of love and appreciation to each part of you. If there's any part of your body that you're unhappy with at the moment, send that area even MORE love and attention.

Say to your body:

I accept you!
I appreciate you so much!
Thank you for everything you did for me yesterday!
Thanks for serving me all night as I sleep.
I love you, darling body.
My beautiful body, each day you get stronger, healthier and more vibrant!
Thank you for everything that you do!
Thank you for being here with me through this lifetime!

In the Bonus section, you will find a white light guided meditation. It's only 7 minutes - use that as a full body refresh whenever you like.

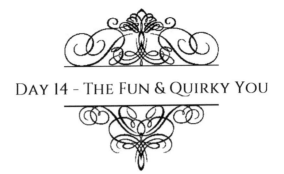

Day 14 - The Fun & Quirky You

10 Fun & Quirky Things You Love About Yourself:

Maybe you like pickles with peanut butter.
Maybe you like telling yourself jokes in the shower.
Your quirks are what make you adorable and unique.

List them!
Ready....go!

T oday, we dip into the fun side of your personality. Reflect on some of the things that are sweet and funny about you. Your little quirks. Did you know that your quirks make you relatable and even more lovable than you already are?

Run your mind through a list of close family and friends and think about which of their quirks make them so special and unique.

Your fun, funny and quirky qualities are simply your unique sparks and ways of processing life. These make you shine with vibrancy and life expression, and are a gift to yourself and others in your life experience.

These are wonderful expressions of your inner joy as you flow along your life path. Enjoy them, celebrate them - they make up the singular uniqueness that is YOU.

There will NEVER be anyone like you in this world!

Advanced Game Play:

- What are some fun quirks of one of your friends?
- Think about a family member – what are their funny and cute quirks?
- How about those of your pet, or a friend's pet?

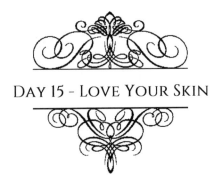

Day 15 - Love Your Skin

10 Things You Love About Your Skin:

Gently touch the skin on the back of your hand.

Your skin protects you and regulates so many body functions.
And on top of that, it's soft and sweet!

What do you love about your skin?
Ready....go!

T oday, you will embrace your skin with attention and love!

Your skin is one of the largest organs in your body. It regulates your body's processes and protects you day and night. Your skin is also the center of sensation.

Take a moment to look down at your arms. Notice the texture of your skin, the hairs, and the shades of color. Gently release any judgement; just look upon this wondrous organ that works with you, for you, day and night.

Gently touch the back of your hand. Feel the sensation of your skin under your fingertips (focus here on the sensation in your fingertips).

Now continue, but switch your attention to the back of your hand and feel the sensation of being touched (this time, focus on the sensation on your hand). In other words, flip to noticing the sensation from both perspectives.

Doesn't that feel lovely?

Advanced Game Play:

Here's an exercise that will change the way you see your skin:

Set aside 5-10 minutes today at home when you will have some privacy.

Undress to the extent that you are comfortable. I suggest stripping entirely.

Once you're ready, gaze down at your skin. Really notice it. You can look at your skin in the mirror as well, if you like.

Again, as in any part of these exercises, if judgements arise, accept them in the moment and release them.

As you gaze at your skin from head to foot, gently run your fingertips down your body. Start from your forehead and run your fingertips around your eyes, down over your nose, trail them over your lips, over your throat and continue like this all the way down your body from your head to your toes.

It may feel very strange the first time or so.

This exercise, however, will unlock the most wonderful appreciation of your skin.

You can use both hands if you like, to gently trail your fingertips over as much of your skin as you please.

It might tickle, and you may find yourself smiling uncontrollably. Our skin was meant to be touched. It loves to be caressed!

As you run your fingertips down your body, send your skin some warm love. You can say out loud:

Thank you, my beautiful skin

I love you!

I love everything you do for me

I love how you protect me

I love how you feel

I love how good it feels when something soft touches you!

I adore the feeling of seaside breezes on you!

I love how the warmth of the sun feels on you.

I love how you serve me day and night, and when I sleep

I love how healthy and firm and vibrant you are!

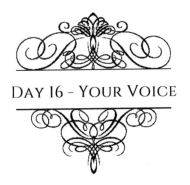

DAY 16 - YOUR VOICE

10 THINGS YOU LOVE ABOUT YOUR VOICE:

Your voice can soothe, or it can emit power.

Your voice can be a lullaby and a ROARRR.

And everything in between.

What do you love about your voice?

Ready....go!

T oday is all about your voice. Your voice is the conduit from your heart to the outer world; it is the connector, the communicator.

Your voice creates and builds relationships using words, and expresses emotions through your tone and energy.

Your voice embodies your emotions when you sing. In fact when you sing, you engage and direct the breath of life through all your organs. Singing transcends time and space. Singing pulls energy into you through a continuous flow of breath, a blending of senses and emotion.

Your voice is not just the sound that comes out of your mouth, it is everything that builds and moves behind it. Your voice is how you express your personality, your ideas, your love, your intentions, your desires, everything.

Your voice carries more power and influence than you can imagine.

Advanced Game Play:

Send love to your throat area with this little exercise...

Visualize a warm golden light, infused with healing vibrations, expanding and growing in your heart area. This light is Love. Simply rest with this for a few moments and then amplify the feeling.

Now gently move this light upwards into your throat area and let it circulate in a clockwise direction.

Imagine the light expanding outwards and filling every nook and cranny in your throat, healing and energizing.

Feel the warmth infusing the path from your heart to your throat.

From this moment onwards, your true intentions and emotions will flow with increasing clarity, confidence and freedom through your voice.

Know that your voice is a gift to yourself and the world around you. See yourself filling your voice with love and light each morning.

If you are a speaker, voice actor or singer – bless and thank your voice. Send it love and gratitude for being your faithful and loving friend and partner.

DAY 17 - FAMILY

FAMILY:

Think about one special family member.
Or someone who is like family to you.

What do you LOVE about them?

What makes them unique and connects
you both together?

Ready....go!

Our closest bonds are formed with family. Our experiences range from having loving and nurturing families all the way through the spectrum to the opposite scenario.

And then there are those beautiful souls who you've met along your life path, people who were there for you and embodied the ideal values within a family – trust, acceptance, unconditional love and affection, mentoring and any other values that are important to you. For me, this treasure trove of family extends to my in-laws as well.

Take a moment now and think back along your life journey. Who did you bond and connect with as family in all the ways that are meaningful to you, whether you are related or not? Think of someone who had the most positive impact on your life.

What is it about that person that you value and cherish?

What was it about them that really connected you both?

What do you love about them?

Advanced Game Play:

If this person is still in your life, consider sending them a handwritten note in a card.

Or perhaps send them an email or give them a call to let them know how much they mean to you.

If they have passed on, write the note anyway and keep it in a journal as a sweet and potent reminder of the beauty and inspiration you received from them. Their energy will live on with you!

DAY 18 - FRIENDS

FRIENDS:

Think about one special friend.

What do you LOVE about them?
What are their wonderful qualities?

Ready....go!

F riends cover such a rich range of connection. Perhaps you have casual friends who are your party buddies - the times are fun and the conversations light and fresh. You may also have friends who are at their best when sharing intimate 1:1 catch ups or engaging in lively discussions.

And then you have friends who are always there for you in all the ways that are meaningful on a deeper level.

Some friends come and go out of your life and yet others can be there with you for a lifetime. Friends are so valuable in their own unique ways, connecting with different aspects of you, and at different stages of your life and situations.

Think about your friends right now.

- Who are you connected to the most in all the ways that make friendship enjoyable?

- What is it about this person that makes them so wonderful and delightful?

- Why do you love spending time with them?

Advanced Game Play:

Contact one of your friends today by phone, text or email and let them know how much you appreciate them.

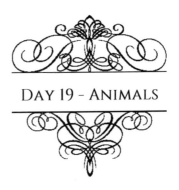

DAY 19 - ANIMALS

ANIMALS:

Think about one of your favourite animals

or pets.

What do you LOVE about them?

What do they signify to you?

A nimals hold a very special connection to humans. Ancient cultures relied on animals for their very lives and many of these cultures held a sacred appreciation for them.

These cultures delved deeply into the characteristics of each animal and imbued mythology and other spiritual practices with their powerful symbolism and meaning.

The appearance of wild animals even now holds deep meaning on a spiritual level for many, and can be considered an energetic message received from the Universe.

In whatever way we individually connect with animals, wild or tame, this connection is one of spirit and mystery. With tame animals such as pets, there is a level of joy that brings vibrancy and life into the present moment.

Here's a little personal story that illustrates the power of the Law of Attraction...

I've been allergic to cats and any animal dander since birth. If I'm around cats or even in a room that was vacated by one, I'd break out in hives and sneeze for hours or days. I've never had a pet, but I always loved the idea of kittens - I mean who doesn't, right? I'd never actually seen kittens in real life (just adult cats), but I adore looking at kitten pictures and videos.

Last year, my youngest daughter begged for a cat. We reminded her that I was allergic and unfortunately couldn't have one. But I started watching kitten videos and actively searching for more online, just for the pleasure of watching. And after a while, I began thinking: *Wouldn't it be so much fun to have a cute kitten? Wouldn't it be amazing to not be allergic?*

Without realizing it, I began to follow all the steps in the manifestation process:

Desire
Focused attention
Visualizing with strong positive emotion
Inspired action (researching types of cats that were the least allergic, for fun)
Non-attachment to the outcome

A year passed and one day my daughter mentioned that her best friend's cat had just delivered a litter of kittens. We were to pick up my daughter from their house that evening. It turned out to be the most wonderful and adorable experience meeting these little babies. I held one and it was so little - it just fit in one hand!

It was only after we left their home that I realized I had completely forgotten to take an antihistamine. But the weird thing was...I had no allergic reaction! We went back again a few more times to see the kittens before they began giving them away – and each time I had no allergy symptoms again. And these were not short-haired cats, they were fluffy!

So, I said to my family: *let's go for it!*

I was a bit worried though...what if it was completely different being close to a cat 24/7 at home? Would I be sneezing the rest of my days away?

Well I'm still amazed to say this, but we've had our kitten for several months as I write this – and not a single allergic reaction in all this time. No matter the reason for the allergy disappearing, I believe I manifested this scenario. And this kitten, this playful, sweet and funny little soul, has brought so much magic into our home.

So...back to you...

- Do you have a pet that is beloved to you?
- How do you love showing affection to your pet and how does your pet show affection to you?
- If you don't have pets, is there a particular animal that holds great meaning and significance for you?
- What emotions do they bring up in you?

Advanced Game Play:

If you have a pet, cuddle him or her in your arms and send warm, love energy from your heart centre. You may feel this as a joyful surge up and outwards.

Look at your pet with your full loving attention, feel them breathing in your arms, feel their texture, their comforting weight in your hands.

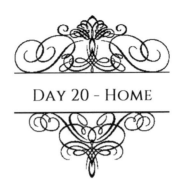

DAY 20 - HOME

HOME:

Home is our cradle, our refuge.

Share 10 things you absolutely LOVE about your home.

Ready....go!

Your home is your safe space, your refuge and your shelter. It's a place where you can create and decorate in ways that soothe and refresh your soul and express your artistic side.

Your bedroom is the womb of your home, a yin space of coziness where you regenerate each day anew. A place of sensual splendor or simplicity – whatever calls to your senses at each stage of your life.

Your kitchen is the yang space of your abode, some say it is the life force, the center of family replenishing and connection.

It's important to note that depending on your current life situation, there may be things about your home that don't appeal to you for certain reasons. It's okay. Allow yourself to accept it. I invite you to try to generate a little love or appreciation for your current home situation as best you can anyway. You can still take steps to have the situation fixed or start the process of focusing on your ideal home. This exercise will allow you to get into a better feeling place now, while also using it as a springboard for change.

If you're at home now, take a little walk around and look for anything that you love. If you're in a place of transition as I just mentioned, or perhaps staying with someone else or in the moving process, acknowledge anything that you love or appreciate there, from the smallest room to any of the items or furnishings.

If you're not at home when you read this, visualize and mentally walk through your home, lingering in front of everything you love.

Make a list of all that you love in your home.
You can do this on paper, in an online document, or even run through a list in your mind.

What do you love about the following?
- Each room
- Your furnishings and fixtures
- Your belongings
- Your decorations
- The location
- The energetic qualities of each space

Advanced Game Play:

In ancient Vedic and Hawaiian spirituality – and confirmed by quantum physics – **everything is energy, both animate and inanimate**.

In Ho'oponopono, a clearing mantra is one of many tools used to help clear old stories, limiting thoughts, old conditioning and old data. The clearing mantra involves 4 specific phrases.
I'm sorry
Please forgive me
Thank you
I love you

From a Ho'oponopono perspective, our mental clutter prevents us from fully experiencing our natural state of love and from truly experiencing the present. All four phrases in this mantra are addressed to the Divine within you to help clear old data and memories out of the present moment. However, the mantra can also be used for anything and for any situation, for living beings or inanimate objects.

The practice of Ho'oponopono is quite deeply layered, so for the purpose of this Game we're going to use the last two phrases only in a very specific way.

Gratitude and **love** are the most powerful emotions to generate from within and to share with others.

Continue to walk around your home, either in person or mentally, and send out your love to each part of your home. In the first part of today's exercise, you appreciated what you *already* love. In the Advanced Game play here, you're consciously sending out love to *every* part of your home.

Say to your home:

Thank you so much, I love you!

I love you, hallway, thank you for welcoming me each day and every time I come home.

I love you living room. Thank you for the cozy space where I can entertain my friends or snuggle up with a wonderful book.

Thank you, my kitchen. Thank you for the space to store and create all the nourishment I need and desire. I love you!

I love you, bathroom. I love you mirror, thank you for letting me see myself in this wonderful miracle of a body.

I love you, shower! You refresh me, thank you so much!

I love you, dining room! I love you, living room! I love you, basement!

Touch your furnishings, your stuff, the walls, the doors, and the windows – whatever you feel inspired to touch. It's okay, no one is watching. Just send *love* to your home, give love – and feel the sensation of powerful loving emotions that begin to surge up and through your body and expand outwards.

It doesn't matter if you have stuff that you want to replace, just give and send love to everything that you have right now.

It will change your life experience in the now moment.

And the *now* is life.

DAY 21 - WORK

WORK:

Work can be tricky.

But it only takes 17 seconds to pivot your

vibrations towards a better feeling direction.

Let's try it.

Think of one of your colleagues. One whom

you admire or connect with.

What do you LOVE about him or her?

Ready....go!

L ife at work is an interesting experience in itself. There are so many preconceived notions and recommendations about how to "be" at work...

How to connect with colleagues, clients, vendors, bosses and more. And for many people, perhaps yourself as well, there may be triggers at work.

Perhaps you come in each day ready and fresh, but ten minutes later you're annoyed and muttering words that rhyme with "puck." (Been there!)

In the manifesting community, there tends to be a little confusion about appreciating the present when there's something unpleasant in it. For example, trying to like your job even if you hate it. The question arises: *if I appreciate this crap, won't I just get more of it because of my attention to it?*

That's a completely understandable point. From an LOA perspective, your current vibration is paving the way to your future experience. So if you can generate some thoughts, words, or feelings of love and appreciation now, you are consciously resetting your path to a better future situation through your mindset.

However, you continue the manifesting process by visualizing your ideal job and taking steps towards it. In these cases, you're training your mind to be at peace with the now, so that you can redirect your focus towards what you do want.

Please know that when it comes to unacceptable experiences that cause pain to yourself or others, I'm not suggesting that we try to turn them into something lovable, or even that we accept them as such.

On the contrary, we can only accept *the experience itself as it has already happened or is unravelling in the present, deal with them in the best way possible* and *then* move with purpose towards what we want, whether that is justice or a new vision.

In this exercise, you're going to focus on what you appreciate in someone at work. Think about the most interesting and inspiring person that you interact with. It doesn't matter what sort of position they have or what they do. Just pick one person you really admire or appreciate.

If you don't work at a traditional day job, use this exercise to think of one particular individual, vendor, client or someone else that you connect with regularly from a business perspective.

Jot down anything and everything you really love about them.

Send thanks mentally to your colleague or associate for being in your life, and for bringing your attention to their inspiring qualities.

Advanced game play:

If you'd like to go a little deeper with this game, think about all the aspects of your job or career that you love. Even if it's just one. And then expand on it. What is that thing that you love about it? Is it your desk, your office, the coffee, the fun laughs?

If you detest your job, think about anything else at all that is desirable there – the pay for example or the location. If it's your pay that you appreciate, think about what your pay brings you, what you do with it and how it affects you.

You can (and should) still look for another job, career or vocation you desire if things are not good, but begin the mindset transformation while you're at your current job.

If you work from home, think about all the wonderful aspects of this. The convenience, perhaps, or the ability to work in your pajamas!

Think about what you can do daily to enhance love and collaboration even more within your workplace. Perhaps you can incorporate them in the way you perform your daily work processes, or in your interactions with your colleagues.

And then mentally walk through your workplace and simply say *I love you, thank you* over and over as you walk around.

As Ho'oponopono master Dr Hew Len says, "You don't have to feel the love when you say it." Just say it anyway, and the love will begin to come.

Day 22 - Surroundings

Surroundings:

Look around your workplace for a minute.

Or, if you're at home, take a peek outside. What do you LOVE about your workplace or street?

Ready....go!

T oday, simply look outside and notice all the things you love and appreciate about your surroundings.

For your home, notice what you like about your garden if you have one, or what you enjoy in your immediate surroundings.

Advanced Game Play:

- What are you situated close to, that you love?

- A park, maybe, where you can relax?

- Or near other enjoyable amenities?

- Or perhaps you enjoy easy access to work?

- What else do you really appreciate in your vicinity?

- If you're at work right now, what is it that you love about the location or the surroundings?

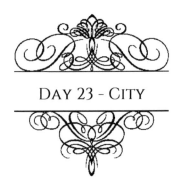

DAY 23 - CITY

CITY:

Your city has its own style, its own pace, a unique energy.

What do you LOVE about your city?

Ready....go!

I n this exercise, I invite you to contemplate the qualities of your city. Although I'm using the word *city,* it can also cover *town* or *village,* depending on where you reside.

- What do you love about your city?

- Is it known for something special and unique?

- What do you love about the energy of your city?

- Where do you love to spend your time in your city?

- What are some of your favorite hang outs?

- Where do you love to walk, to drive, to bike, to sit?

Advanced Game Play:

Search for your city on Wikipedia. Or Google "the best of (your city name)." For fun, read through everything you find.

Then send out love and appreciation to all who have made your city a very special place...

- Whoever designed and built your streets.

- Those who planted trees and who take care of the city landscaping.

- The people who clean the streets.

- The owners and clerks who operate the stores that you love to visit.

- The restaurants and the people who cook the meals you love, those who serve you, and the ones who clean.

- The engineers who designed your transit system. The bus and subway operators.

- Your city support system that fixes everything, or those who remove the garbage.

- Those who designed, built and operate your community services. The pools, the classes, the gyms, the parks.

- The hospitals and medical offices in your city.

- The hotels, the sports and concert stadiums and places of leisure.

- The cozy spaces that you love.

- The artists that bring imagination, design, colour and beauty to your senses.

- The musicians that bring your city to life.

- And anyone else that comes to mind – you'll think of more each time you play!

To anything and everything in your city - just say: *Thank you, I love you!*

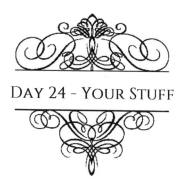

DAY 24 - YOUR STUFF

STUFF!

Look around your home or your office.

Everything is energy...

Which of your material possessions do you LOVE?

Ready....go!

There's no shame in loving your stuff. Just because they're material items, it doesn't make them unworthy of love.

There's a saying you may have heard before: *Love people. Use things. Not the other way around.*

I'd tweak that to: *Love people. Love your stuff. But love people more!*

In this game play, look around your workspace or your home. Look for anything you own, that you love.

If you're at work when you read this, do the exercise at work, then do it again when you get home.

Advanced Game Play:

Physically touch your stuff. Touch the things in your office, the items in your rooms at home.

Gently touch the clothes in your closets, your coats, your shoes, your clothing in drawers, your curtains.

Trail your hand lightly over all your things as you walk from room to room.

As you do so, just say:

Thank you, I love you for being with me!
Thank you for letting me play with you!
Thank you for being part of my home and my life!
Thank you, I love you!

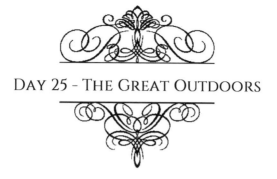

DAY 25 - THE GREAT OUTDOORS

THE GREAT OUTDOORS:

What do you LOVE about nature?
A certain flower? Trees? Mountains? The
ocean?

What nature-filled magnificence makes
you feel wonderful?

List as many as you can think of!
Ready....go!

I n this game play, consider all the aspects of nature that you love.

This can be anything you love *about* nature itself, or what you love to *experience in* nature.

Mountains, trees, lakes, beaches, sand, islands, flowers - what do you love about them and which call out to your soul in a special way?

The elements of nature – what type of weather do you love and which are your favorite seasons?

How about wild animals – which bring out the wonder in you?

Advanced Game Play:

- Which cities, places and countries are you drawn to?

- What is it about each of them that fascinate you?

- Which would you love to visit in person?

- Which place would you love to visit first?

Google everything you can about the place you'd love to visit first on your list and open a folder on your desktop. For extra fun, see if you can find a Facebook group dedicated for lovers of that city or location, and join it.

Search for anything about this location that inspires you, including flight or travel costs to get there, best hotel reviews, restaurants, sightseeing and other things to enjoy. Save these links. Open a Word document and add your own notes. They'll come in handy one day!

Save pictures to your desktop, or place into a digital vision board (a simple Word document or your desktop will work fine).

Most importantly, **revel in the feelings.** Feel that you're enjoying this trip in the here and now, as you're going through all the research online.

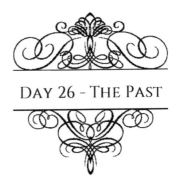

DAY 26 - THE PAST

THE PAST:

Think back a little...

What are some of the things - or who are some of the people - in your past, that have made you the amazing person you are today?

List as many as you can think of!
Ready....go!

I n this exercise, you're going to mentally take a little journey through your past and think about certain events and people who've helped co-create the wonderful person you are today.

What are some of the most exciting and wonderful events that make up your life story?

Who are some of the people in your past that really contributed to your personal growth and values? It's perfectly fine if this overlaps with earlier exercises in the Game, it's part of the fun!

Advanced Game Play:

- What are some of your best memories?

- What's one of the best decisions you've ever made?

- What are some of the best concerts or shows you can remember attending?

- What are some of the most fun times you've had till now?

- What are some of the best vacations you've been on?

- What did you do last month that was awesome?

- How about last week?

- What did you do or experience yesterday that was wonderful?

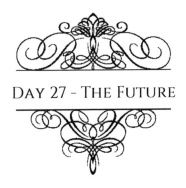

Day 27 - The Future

The Future:

What are you SO looking forward to:

Next week?

Next month?

Next year?

List them all!

Ready...go!

I f we truly knew what the future would bring, we'd all have won the lottery by now. The truth is that although you can attempt to predict, plan and schedule things, life happens in the moment and anything can change, most especially if your focus and desires change as well. And that's okay.

Life was meant to have the element of change.

Since you don't know for sure what's going to happen in the future, why not imagine the best possibilities ahead for you?

- What are you looking forward to in the near future?

- Who are you looking forward to seeing soon?

- Which events, get-togethers, concerts and other upcoming activities are you really excited about?

Advanced Game Play:

1. Make a list by *week*, *month* and *year* of your upcoming events and save them in an email draft or in a document.

2. Create a separate list called *To Book*.

3. Add upcoming ideas, concerts and trips to the *To Book* document.

4. Add dates to your Calendar to remind yourself to take action on the *To Book* items, or to take the next inspired action step towards them.

5. Add them into your budget.

6. Add to your lists whenever new events get booked.

By the way, don't add any appointment that you're not really excited about onto these lists. Keep them in your scheduler instead. These lists are only for enjoyable events and dates.

Each time you look at your lists, you'll feel anticipation and excitement!

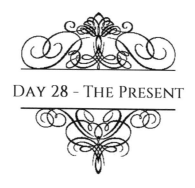

DAY 28 - THE PRESENT

THE PRESENT:

THIS....is your moment of power.

Take a look around you.

Glance down at your hands, your body, your surroundings.

Breathe deeply for a minute.

What do you LOVE about this very moment?

Ready....go!

I f our present is built upon certain events, experiences and a mindset from the past, then the future takes root from our experiences, mindset, responses and thoughts that spring from this moment.

By now, you have likely realized that every single exercise you've been playing here is all about the moment of "now."

No matter where you've been mentally or physically while playing, it's always been happening **now – you're playing *now*** - even if envisioning the past or future.

This moment is the most wonderful and exciting moment of all – it is the seed for the next moment, your future experiences and your future life.

Look around at where you are right now and simply feel the energy. Feel into this space.
Look down at your body right now. You'll never be as young as you are now in linear time, so enjoy it!

Be exquisitely aware of this moment. It is unfolding in front of you – FOR you.
Touch your hands, feel your face. You are **alive**!

Every possibility for your future lies in this very moment.
It lies in your attention, your clarity and your focus.
It lies in your intentions, your purpose, your hopes, your dreams and goals.

Dreams and goals transition into your real-life creations as you focus upon them with consistency and clarity. And they flow with momentum with your actions.

Manifesting is attention, so give your attention to what you want to have more of in your life.

Advanced Game Play:

Be aware of where your attention goes in your present moment.

Choose where you want to direct your attention and gently withdraw it from anything that doesn't serve you. Deal with those situations, of course, as best as you can – then quickly turn your attention to what you want.

Thank you and *I love you* are the greatest of all mantras – prayers - to your inner Divinity, embraced within all Universal Energy. These two phrases are the most profound bridges that connect you to everything and everyone in your life.

Thank you for playing through the 28 Days.

Thank you for giving yourself the attention you truly deserve.

The *Law of Attraction*

GAME BOOK

28 DAYS OF

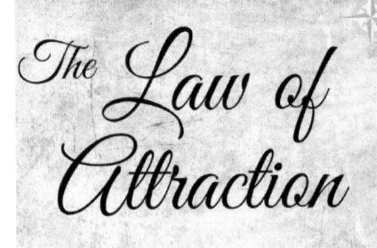

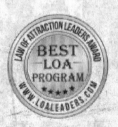

THE DAILY
POWER RITUAL

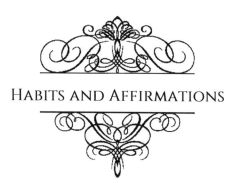

HABITS AND AFFIRMATIONS

During this Game, you've been on a wonderful journey to re-discover how unique and amazing you are!

You've created a daily habit that gives attention to positive aspects about yourself and your life.

But maybe you're wondering: *Well now what? How do I make this last? How do I make this my new normal?*

Have you ever heard of the saying that it takes approximately 21 days to change or set up a new habit? This is a misquote that snowballed over the years. James Clear mentions something fascinating in his book *Atomic Habits*: It actually takes a *minimum* of 21 days to form a new habit.

Research shows that **it actually takes *an average* of 66 days for a new habit to develop**. And the best part is that it's fine if you fall off the wagon and forget to practice your new habit for a day or two occasionally. As long as you continue the new habit for the duration for the 66 days, even if off and on, the habit will integrate into your lifestyle.

I chose 28 days for this Game so we could surpass the 21-day minimum. Now we're going to kick things up a notch to the next level of 66 days in an incredibly fun and easy way.

We humans have a habit of rounding up or rounding down numbers. So instead of 66 days which is just a little over 2 months, we're going to incorporate this practice into a 90-day cycle. Easy to plan, easy to remember and easy to implement.

In this section, you're going to create a simple but powerful daily ritual. It's a ritual that will serve as an easy tool – it's a way to appreciate yourself on an ongoing basis. **Done consistently and daily, you will create an internal robust powerhouse of expanding self-worth.**

Do this for 90 days and not only will it reset your daily mindset, but it will transform you through a conscious and external dimension into the inner cellular dimension. You will quite literally be rewiring yourself for success by expanding your self-confidence from a newfound position of self-worth.

We're going to be ramping up the momentum. Newton's First Law of Motion brings this concept to life: "An object at rest stays at rest and an object in motion stays in motion with the same speed and in the same direction unless acted upon by an unbalanced force." In this case, we're using the daily ritual to boost the force in the direction that you want to go.

After we explore the basics of the ritual, we're going to look at different types of "believers." You will have fun discovering which type of believer resonates with you the most - and more importantly how the Daily Power Ritual will satisfy *any* type of believer on a conscious and subconscious level.

You'll need to set aside a little uninterrupted time for this exercise, so come back to this section when you have some privacy. Considering how powerful this Ritual is, the more time you allow yourself to create it, the better.

You'll need your notebook, a pen, and the answers from your daily Games.

You can also type the upcoming exercises into a document if you prefer that to a notebook.

Ready?

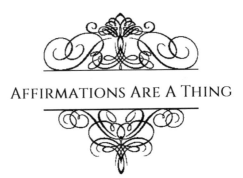

AFFIRMATIONS ARE A THING

Have you ever thought that an affirmation seems a bit like a fake wanna-be statement? That it might be a way to try and fool yourself into believing something that isn't true?

I used to think that way a lot. I used to ask myself; *how does it* work *for those people? It's not even remotely close to being true for me! How am I supposed to state something if it seems completely unbelievable? I feel stupid saying this.*

Yes, I was quite skeptical of affirmations. Until the day I realized something that you've probably also realized...**we are *constantly* affirming something - either negative, neutral or positive every single day**, often all day long. Sometimes we affirm things about ourselves and other times we affirm with regards to other people, things, or situations.

Affirming is the process of stating something as though it is true. Our conscious mind is in the process of agreeing with the content of our thoughts or with our verbal statements.

We normally affirm in a very simple and general manner.

Some examples of negative affirmations...

So-and-so is really annoying!

My stomach looks so fat!

This bus is late again.

That guy is always so negative (the irony, haha!)

Some examples of neutral affirmations...

I'm making nachos tonight.

It's sunny outside.

My new headphones arrived today.

I own that blue Honda Civic over there.

Some examples of positive affirmations...

I'm actually kind of fun and funny!

He takes such good care of our family.

I always look great in that color!

She's so kind to people.

Notice how the affirmation tense is either in the past, present or future. But no matter what tense or timeline is used, the affirmations themselves are usually simple statements worded as fact.

Affirmation secret: It's easier to believe – and therefore to assimilate – a simply worded statement.

If you've already used affirmations consciously as a tool for either personal growth or manifesting, have you had varying degrees of success? Have they worked sometimes, but not at other times?

Along with simplicity in the way it's worded, the *potency* of an affirmation and whether or not it manifests into your life depends on your belief structure:

- what type of believer you are in general, or with regards to a specific desire
- the "believability" of each affirmation

Later we'll look at a few types of believers. First, we'll create your Super Affirmations, and then you'll be able to see how they fit into *any* belief structure without effort.

CREATING YOUR SUPER AFFIRMATIONS

G rab your notebook, pen (or open a Word document) and have handy all your answers from the 28 Days of Love Playsheets.

For an example, pull out the answers for Day 9 – what you love about your laugh.

Create your first Super Affirmation by combining all your answers for Day 9 together into one present-tense statement, beginning with "I love", "I am" or "I have." To do that, read through the qualities you came up with earlier and notice which ones make you feel the best when you read them.

You may feel a surge of pleasure straight from the navel. Or you may feel warm and smiley. Place those qualities closer to the beginning of your Super Affirmation. That will start off each affirmation with a real boost!

Let's do an example together:

Original answers...

My laugh is attractive.

My laugh is musical.

My laugh is so heartfelt (1)

My laugh is fun (3)

It's warm (2)

It's funny

My laugh is easy

It's engaging

My laugh is catchy

It's also kind of sassy!

Step 1:
Read through your answers and jot down a number from 1-10 next to each answer, 1 being the most pleasurable when you think about it. I've placed numbers 1 to 3 as an example above.

Step 2:
Start creating your Super Affirmation, using *I am, I have or I love*, and add on your qualities from 1 to 10, in that order.

Using the example above:

I LOVE how my laugh is so heartfelt, warm, fun, funny, easy, attractive, engaging, musical, catchy and sassy!

It's short, (short for 10 qualities!) simple, and in the present tense. But most importantly, you already believe every word of yours!

Here's an example for Day 10 – what you love about yourself, using a slightly different structure:

I am loving, friendly, supportive, smart, creative, lovely, a great friend, I'm a loving daughter, I'm LOADS of fun and I have a great sense of humor!

See how easy it is to tweak into a simple statement?

Now take a little time to create each of yours from Day 1 to 28.

Some of the Days have longer answers – use your creativity to hone and summarize, hone down again and clarify the answers to their best, clearest and shortest forms.

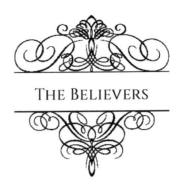

THE BELIEVERS

B elief in a desire, a dream, and a goal – believing in anything or anyone is a necessary part of the manifestation process. It's the one aspect that can halt or speed up manifestation of either a physical experience, or a character trait.

Belief is an energetic investment in something or someone.

Below are a few types of believers – perhaps you may relate to some or all of these. Or maybe you find yourself one type of believer under certain situations and conditions, yet another type of believer for something else.

You may also notice that you've experienced each type of belief before, like signposts along your life path – from a more disempowered state to one of increased self-confidence.

Along with each type of believer is a suggested root from which these manifest, along with why your Super Affirmations will work for this type of believer.

The Dis-Believer:

You experience certain desires and affirmations manifesting, but you still feel like they're not quite real, or that they're too good to be true and will disappear from your life. Or you doubt that you really had the personal clout to manifest them – therefore their appearance in your life must be a coincidence.

Root: Fear from having losses in the past and a fear of being disappointed in the future.

Super Affirmations: You already know that the content in your Super Affirmations are a part of you, a part of your personality, and your history. You *know* they are real. So there's no wishful thinking happening with the Super Affirmation that you could ever lose out on later.

I'll Believe It When:

You're a lover of your senses, and practical. You believe something only when you experience it for yourself, or after manifesting it into your life.

Root: Your dreams and desires may have been ridiculed by others in the past, leading to a lack of confidence in the unseen becoming manifest.

Super Affirmations: All the statements that you're affirming have already manifested in one way or another – which is why you were able to come up with them in the Game. And since they already exist, they have manifested for you.

I'll Believe It Because She / He Said So:

You trust the opinion of certain trendsetters, icons or experts in their fields. You also place weight on reviews and testimonials, all of which appear to lend credibility to something you want to be, do or have. You believe others when they say something about your appearance, skills or personality. You also doubt the possibilities of manifesting something you want unless you have support from others.

Root: Your dreams and desires may have been squashed by others in authority long ago resulting in a lack of confidence in your own opinions, and your adventurous spirit being limited and curtailed.

Super Affirmations: One of the Days celebrates what others already say about you. And the answers for the rest of the Days are based upon your own knowledge of what's lovable about you. That's content from 27 days out of 28 that YOU know to be 100% true of yourself – from within you. That's personal power.

I'll Believe It Because I Must:

You've been trained or raised with certain ideas about what's possible for you. Or perhaps the idea of *not* believing in something or someone would be painful to you. You might not be sure exactly *why* you believe in something, only that you do.

Root: Certain paths have been laid out for you by others resulting in a dependency on authority figures or a fixed belief system.

Super Affirmations: You played this Game because you wanted to, not because you needed to. You didn't choose the things that are lovable about yourself because you *had* to, you chose them because you know they're true already. You discovered your own responses to the Game, you're creating your own Super Affirmations & Ritual just the way you please. That's personal power too.

The Optimistic Believer:

You're not sure if what you believe or affirm is true or will come to pass, but you believe in *hope,* and you want it so badly that you'll focus on your hope again and again even through the rough times.

Root: You have a strong desire for things to be different, but lack of clarity on exactly what you want to be, do and have.

Super Affirmations: What you noticed about yourself in your daily statements and in your affirmations are completely clear. They are what they are. You don't have to *hope* you have those qualities or that you manifested certain things into your life. You *know* you have those qualities. You *did* those things already. They are all part of your life story.

The Confident Believer:

You feel a certainty from within that what you're affirming is either true now in some way, or will definitely manifest into your life. Perhaps you may have already started seeing physical proof of a desire. Or if you haven't manifested a desire or an affirmation yet, either your doubts have decreased or your self-confidence has increased to the point where you *know* they will manifest with time - you're willing to wait it out and keep your focus and inspired action steady.

Root: You've built up your inner strength from perceived mistakes in your past. You have clarity and focus.

Super Affirmations: You are aligned with your affirmations and you know they are all part of the flow. You realize that the ebbs are also a natural part of flow, and you can move with it now with much more ease than in the past.

Habit-izing, Creating and Automating Your Daily Power Ritual

N ow we're going to seamlessly connect everything into your Daily Power Ritual.

According to James Clear, *the best way to break a bad habit is to make it impossible to do. And the best way to create a good habit is to automate it so you never have to think about it again.*

Time and energy vampires are the biggest detriments to manifesting what you want. Take a clear look at your daily lifestyle and give yourself permission to limit or stop anything that sucks away your time and energy that isn't in alignment with your chosen lifestyle. This sounds rather lofty but it can be a challenge to put into practice! Like with anything – just do your best. And always be kind to yourself.

I suggest to minimize the following 2 general habits for the full duration of your 90 days. You'll see immediate improvements to where you spend your time which is incredibly empowering. And limiting these may positively affect your mood in a wonderful way (they did mine, and all the other players in the live Game).

1. Pick a one-hour time slot (or 2 x 30 min) for social media daily and use only that time to browse, read and post. Stay logged out of social media for the rest of the day and night.

2. Reduce or completely stop watching, reading or listening to the news. If you want to stay in the news-loop, choose your stories selectively. If you must do it, reduce your news time to 5 minutes a day.

Now we're going to set up and automate your Daily Power Ritual so it's effortless and you don't have to think about it.

Creating Your Daily Power Ritual:

This is the easiest part of the Game!

Collect all your Super Affirmations and put them together on one page. You'll have 28 lines of power statements, and all of them you KNOW are true!

First write them line by line onto a sheet of paper (or in a lovely notebook). You should end up with 1 or 2 pages of written Super Affirmations.

Now type them line by line into an email. In the subject line, type in the title DAILY POWER RITUAL. Save that email as a draft, we'll get back to it later.

Automating the Daily Power Ritual:

Step 1:

Choose one "automation" method below and stick to it for the duration of the 90 days.

1. Physical and tactile locations (stickies, notebooks, etc.)
2. Online reminders
3. Both

I personally use #3 both. A notebook is a great physical and visual reminder of my affirmations when I want something tactile, but I depend on the online reminders as they're completely automatic. If you have a variety of lovely notebooks available, it's fun to grab whichever one catches your eye in the moment whenever you feel like writing out your Super Affirmations.

In an upcoming Law of Attraction Game Book, I will show you how to set up a daily writing practice that yields incredible manifestation results.

But in this Game, once you have created your Super Affirmations, the reminder is automated and the daily practice will be reading and listening. No more writing needs to be done, unless you choose to do it.

Step 2:

You will be reading your Super Affirmations every day for 90 days (or listening to them if you record them – we'll get to that soon). In this step, we're going to set up your automated reminders.

Physical and tactile reminders:

For a few minutes, think your way through your daily routine. What are your early morning habits after you wake up? What's your daily routine like? Think of places and times when it would be easy for you to notice physical triggers.

Now think of one time in your day when you KNOW you'll have 5 minutes to yourself (even if it's in the bathroom!). This is where you're going to leave a physical copy of your Super Affirmations.

This is also where you want to be highly practical. For example, even though it's often recommended to visualize or do manifesting work upon awakening and right before sleep, if you're usually in a huge rush in the mornings or have a busy routine right before going to sleep, it wouldn't be practical to leave your Super Affirmations next to the bed.

Remember, you don't need to change your routine for this particular automation. What we're doing instead is inserting a new and desired mindset and self-awareness into your **already existing** daily schedule, so that it can be truly automated efficiently into your lifestyle.

I leave all my affirmations in a notebook in my desk at home. I know I'm going to sit there each day at some point or other and it's easy to flick through and read them. I tried the bedside table routine, but my morning and bedtime schedule was so crazy busy that I didn't make time for it. I through about the bathroom routine, but I don't like my affirmations to be read by anyone else. So in this exercise, find what works best for you – what will be more fun - and then incorporate it!

Keep your Super Affirmations Audio (see Advanced Game Play below) in a very visible spot on your smartphone and pick a time of day when you can listen to it, even if it's just playing in the background while you go for a walk or do other things. I listen to mine when I'm walking.

Online Reminders:

If you spend part of your day online, then this is an ideal way to automate your Super Affirmations.

1. First, pick an online Calendar program that includes a reminder feature. I use Google Calendar.

2. Open your email drafts and select the Daily Power Ritual email with all your Super Affirmations that you created earlier.

3. On a separate window, open a new Calendar item. Name it "DAILY POWER RITUAL - read me!" or something else that you like.

4. Now copy and paste all your Super Affirmations from your email draft into the description body of your Calendar reminder.

5. Include a link to the Super Affirmation Audio, if possible, at the bottom of the description.

6. Pick a time of day that you're usually online and available.

7. Set up the Calendar reminder alert for that time of day, and make sure it's set up as a Repeat, for Daily.

8. Toggle the Notification and Email reminders if your Calendar has those features, so that you receive an alert through your email or phone.

Now, each time you receive the automated email or phone alert, you'll be able to open it and read all your Super Affirmations in the body of the email reminder!

Advanced Game Play:

The power of SOUND is indisputable. Music, words, audio, all unleash a level of connection that is different from reading and writing. Record yourself reading your Super Affirmations and save that on your smartphone or computer to listen to each day. You can listen while going for a walk, or sitting at your desk - anytime at all.

1. Download any high-rated free Voice Recorder app onto your smart phone.

2. Do a sample test so you can get the hang of recording a short snippet of yourself speaking. Save the file and listen to it. Email it to yourself as well and get comfortable with it.

3. Look for a piece of music you LOVE. Don't worry about whether it's the "right type" or not. Whatever makes you feel great when you listen to it is the right type! It can be Buddha bar lounge music, spa relaxation, devotional mantras, pop, classical, heavy metal, whatever rocks you out. Pick a tune that pushes your fun energy button.

4. Now play the music through speakers while recording on your smartphone using the Voice Recorder app. Allow a bar or two of the music to play, and then record yourself over the music voicing your Super Affirmations. Have fun with this!

5. Save the clip, listen back, and re-record as needed, adjusting the music volume level so that you have the best mix between your voice and the music.

6. Save your Super Affirmations Audio on a spot on your smartphone or computer where you can easily listen to it daily.

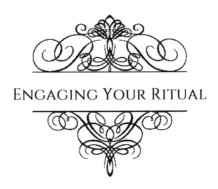

ENGAGING YOUR RITUAL

Here's what you're engaging with the Daily Power Ritual: I've used Jack Canfield's emotional touchpoints below to illustrate how powerful and magical this practice is:

Heart – all your Super Affirmations have been created from your heartfelt daily responses to the Game and you KNOW them to be true already. They've bypassed your belief system alerts because of that fact.

Emotions – you've organized the quality of each Super Affirmation according to your emotions - YOU have determined what works. Remember, you can always change up any part of the affirmations whenever you want. The Audio will also engage you emotionally as you've connected it to a piece of music that heightens your good feelings.

Awareness – using the Law of Attraction, each time you read your Super Affirmations, you become both consciously and subconsciously aware of your high worth.

The daily practice also brings your qualities into your present awareness.

Imagination – you've engaged the energy and vibration of "like attracts like". It becomes easier to recognize your qualities and imagine using them in a positive way. This attracts even more similar thoughts that expand outwards, bringing in more loving desires and loving experiences to imagine based on self-love.

Intuition – as the qualities in your Super Affirmations begin to really settle themselves into your very being each day, your ability to easily recognize them in yourself without conscious reasoning increases.

Physical – everything is energy, so too the way your mind works affects your body. It's easy to pinpoint how your body reacts when you're feeling terrible about something. On the flip side, when you're thinking about your positive qualities on a regular and consistent basis, this mental energy transposes into feelings of wellbeing and a physical demeanor of self-confidence. Consistent feelings of wellbeing will affect your physical body.

Your Will - reading your Super Affirmations as a priority for 90 days – in fact committing to *any* desired activity for 90 days - is a sign that you're using your will in an empowered way for your own benefit!

Higher Self – everything you created in this Game links you to your Higher Self. You embody ALL these beautiful and wondrous qualities. And you DESERVE to remind yourself of your worth! Your Higher Self knows this and adores you!

Once you have strengthened your sense of self-worth, it becomes easier and easier to respond to anything that comes up in your life with your own opinions and using your own judgement.

This in turn transforms your natural flow into clear focus on where you want to *go*, who you want to *be*, and what you want to *have* in your life. It becomes easier and easier to commit to taking inspired action on these with authenticity.

At the end of the 90 days, I suggest that you continue your Daily Power Ritual for as long as you like.

WRAP UP PARTY

Y ou made it to the end of the Game, WOO HOO!!! Congratulations, my friend! If you made it this far, you are truly on the path to inner success!

Anytime you need a massive self-love boost, simply open any version of this Game wherever you are, and play.

Set up a Calendar reminder to play this game again every few months or at least each January for an amazing recharge to the New Year.

You have given yourself the time to dive deep and shine light on your beautiful, playful qualities - and your life.

You've created Super Affirmations that link various aspects of you into powerful and truthful statements.

And you've minimized your availability to the "societal noise" out there, dedicating the time to yourself so you can experience life unfolding from your own unique perspective.

You've created a Daily Power Ritual and you've automated it in a way that you can read or listen to your Ritual each day, with minimum effort.

Your final task:

Set up a Calendar reminder for the conclusion of the 90 days after having started your Daily Ritual.

Think of a rewarding experience that you'd really love...a night out for a rock concert? A night in to read a good book? Dinner out with friends? A weekend away or a vacation?

Pick something that feels fabulous, and as soon as you reach the 90 days, celebrate by booking your experience!

PRINTABLE PLAYSHEETS & BONUSES, WOO HOO!

E njoy the included bonuses – each of them have been lovingly crafted and offered to help you.

1. The Law of Attraction Goal Planner LoveSheet – An Excel spreadsheet set up for you to add your Game Plays, inspired and creative ideas and your Power Ritual.

2. All About Love audio with Marc Allen – listen in on an incredibly inspiring and fun conversation where the award winning author, and publisher of New World Library contemplates the universal nature of Love.

3. Love Guided Meditation – play this guided audio when you go for a walk and feel Love energize your body, mind and spirit.

To download your bonuses, visit

https://www.joyfullifemastery.com/28daysoflove

If you need help to access the download page,

simply email us at JoyfulLifeMastery@gmail.com.

THANK YOU!

E ach time you play this Game, you will intensify the quality of love for yourself - as you should. Your life carries great meaning and wonder!

Each day, you will reveal more of your superpowers to yourself and to the world.

It is my greatest wish that you share all the love that you have to offer with the world in your own unique way - all of which contributes to this powerful Universal creative energy.

May you shine your light bright and strong, beautiful soul!

With love,
Priya

If you enjoyed the Game and believe that others will enjoy it, please share a simple blurb online or send us an email at JoyfulLifeMastery@gmail.com.

Because this will help potential players decide whether the Game could be of value for them. And because your opinion matters.

Thank you, I really appreciate it!

GRATITUDE

To Ken, Janaki and Sundari for everything that matters.

To Nina, Ramesh and Kavita for your enduring love, wisdom and support.

To the dear families that mean so much to me: the Khajuria family, the Davies family and the Alldis family.

To Ken Davies, Rob Onyskiw, Len Balas, and Craig Smith for all the fun times and juicy tunes.

To Asha Frost, Marissa Stapley, Sylvia Pantic, Kit Daven, Andrew Alldis, Philippa Settels, Don Pinkerton, Amisha Modi, Mildred Dias, Tracy Childress, Brian and Michelle Greene, Bob Crisp, Randy Wisebrod, Shazz Carrington, Kiran Sharma, Rob

Ralph, Joyce & Ray Edge and the rest of my wonderful friends and colleagues for your love, friendship and support.

To all the beautiful lightworkers out there, who give and inspire even more love.

To my Sai sisters and brothers who embody truth, goodness and beauty.

To Esther-Hicks and Abraham, Joshua and Gary Bodley, Sanaya Roman and Duane Packer, Laurel and Hope Bradford, all of whom brighten my life.

To Rhonda Byrne, Frederick Dodson, Marc Allen, Deepak Chopra, Louise Hay, Jack Canfield, Brian Tracy, Bob Proctor, Mike Dooley, Joe Vitale, Jeannette Maw, Lisa Marie Hayes, James Clear, Sam Ovens, Elizabeth Purvis, Vishen Lakhiani, Ramit Sethi, Pam Grout, Katrina Ruth and all the wonderful and prolific self-development, Law of Attraction authors, creators and teachers who have influenced and inspired me.

To the incredible love and life coaches in the GoodVibe Coaches League, for maintaining the highest standards of integrity and love for all whom you serve. And for shining light onto the gifts of all who you come across.

To Nonon Tech & Design for your fabulous formatting and editing expertise. And to my Law of Attraction community, for playing these Games and inspiring me every single day.

ABOUT PRIYA KHAJURIA

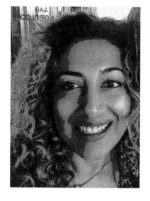

Priya Khajuria creates the award-winning Law of Attraction Games & Adventures that help readers create and live their best life.

She is an author, a voice artist, a Ho'oponopono practitioner, a Law of Attraction coach and has a Bachelors in Psychology. Priya is the lead singer for Peace of Night and the former singer for La La La Human Steps.

Priya's articles have been featured in Vitality Magazine, Think Simple Now, Medium, Positively Positive and Mike Dooley's TUT Blog.

Sign up for the Newsletter and receive a Manifesting Gift Pack:

http://tinyurl.com/yyykdouo

It includes:

- Manifesting freebies
- Goal setting blueprints
- Free VIP membership. Receive early news on Joyful Life Mastery book and product launches, free manifesting Games and more.

www.JoyfulLifeMastery.com

44933651R00091

Made in the USA
Middletown, DE
11 May 2019